# Curing
# Acid Reflux

## Discover the vital link with Breathing

Bala Mookoni

# DISCLAIMER

This book is designed to advise on a healthy lifestyle that assists in curing acid reflux naturally and is not a substitute for proper professional medical advice. As every situation is unique, please consult your doctor before changing the dosage of your medicines.

*I am present in the body as the fiery acid in the stomach. Balancing inhalation and exhalation, I digest the four types of food.*

- Bhagavad Gita, 15:14

# DEDICATION

This is for you, Riya.

# CONTENTS

# 1 INTRODUCTION

Acid reflux is a very common disease in modern times. Drugs treating heartburn from acid reflux, also known as GERD or Gastro Esophageal Reflux Disease, are amongst the highest selling drugs in the world. Yet people who suffer from acid reflux appear to be condemned for a lifetime of medicine for this condition. Apart from the money spent on them, what is of more concern is that these drugs, despite being some of the safest drugs, may have many silent side effects on prolonged use.

When used for a short period, PPIs can be a boon to people with severe, uncontrolled acid reflux. But I have personally known people who had developed severe bone health issues due to extended use of PPIs. Further, some studies indicate a link between PPI usage and memory loss and Alzheimer's disease. There is also a risk of stomach cancer, though current studies indicate this risk is low. All the different drugs used for treating acid reflux do provide relief, in a way that cannot, it appears, be matched by any another method or line of therapy, but they do not address the underlying root causes of the condition. The result is a dependency on the drug and the side effects due to prolonged usage. Moreover, the relief is short term, specific to heartburn, and rarely provides permanent relief to other associated problems such as flatulence, bloating and ulcers.

However, I do strongly recommend modern drugs, especially PPIs, for short-term treatment of and immediate relief from uncontrolled acid reflux, as prolonged untreated acid reflux can cause erosion and damage to the esophagus. By following the methods in this book, the symptoms of acid reflux can subside, and then the usage of drugs should gradually be stopped. Depending on the existing conditions, by following the practices illustrated here, it will be possible to decrease medication in 1-2 weeks' time. But as most people find it difficult to sustain the regime, especially where it involves managing their emotions, an occasional pill may continue to be required to manage that odd incidence of acid reflux on a bad day or after an eating binge. However, at that level, the risk of side effects decreases dramatically. Even in stubborn cases, following the simple methods prescribed here on a regular basis will eventually pave the way for a near-complete, if not complete, cure of acid reflux.

As a Life Coach, I work on various problems people face, and particularly those that are rather intractable to a solution or a cure capture my attention and interest. My work largely revolves around mapping traditional wisdom with modern research and discoveries and coming up with some new (and often startling) correlations. In particular, I delve into the largely undiscovered treasures that lie hidden in the wisdom of mystics that has found expression in the various works of Yoga. Besides, I had personally suffered from acid reflux (that had its onset during prolonged years of shift-working) for nearly a decade. The practices that I have described in this book have worked wonders for me, and I am a living testimony to their efficacy.

In this book, we will see how we can overcome, with minimal changes in our diet, the various problems and discomforts associated with acid reflux and cure the reflux without medicines. I promise you that there will be no fad diets or the introduction of rare and exotic foods. The cures are easily available in everyday life and everyone can do them.

For one, it is now clear that there are no foods or diets that can truly cure acid reflux. It is true that some foods do worsen the condition while some others are more soothing on the stomach. But there is no diet that can cure acid reflux completely or permanently. So, in short, there is neither medicine nor food that can cure acid reflux. There are only palliatives. People who are suffering with acid reflux will vouch for this.

There are any number of books and articles in the market claiming to cure acid reflux through diet, secret foods, exotic natural herbs, ayurvedic medicine, homeopathy, yoga etc. There is no doubt that all these are aimed at improving general health, and, therefore, they do help to some extent. And I recommend most of them to that extent. But if you are looking for that magical cure, that silver bullet or quick fix, something else is required. The reason for this is that ailments related to the digestive system require a different approach.

# 2 UNRAVELLING THE MYSTERY

When the success rate of a solution to a problem is low, we can reasonably be sure that we are not spot on. Some results could appear because of some general benefits. But when the solution has low repeatability, we have to search elsewhere for a fix that lasts and fits for most cases.

In the wisdom of Yoga, the digestive function is affected by the mind-body-spirit (MBS) complex. Therefore, only an approach that works on all the three aspects of this complex has a chance to cure chronic acid reflux. To drive a nail into the wall you have to strike it on its head. To cure the disease of acid reflux we have to engage that single lever that is most capable of working on the MBS complex. Yoga has provided clues to this singular lever.

Today, it is increasingly recognized that several diseases (if not all) have a connection with the mind. While medical science refers to such diseases as psychosomatic disease, Yoga looks at it differently.

Diseases primarily have their origin in emotions and thinking patterns (the Mind in the MBS complex). From there, it percolates down to the physical level, to the physical causes and effects (the Body part in the MBS complex). While the Mind aspect is a response to an external stimulus (in the form of various thoughts and emotions), per Yoga there is a subconscious intelligence in our bodies that not only regulates our autonomic nervous system but also controls our innate tendencies, traits and physical faculties. In a simplistic model, let us call this subconscious intelligence as the Spirit. The Spirit can neither been seen with eyes nor be known by touch. So, how can we work on something that can neither be seen nor be touched? Again, traditional Yoga provides an answer: **Balanced Breathing**. The working of the Spirit can be regulated through breathing techniques.

The three pillars of the MBS complex are intertwined. Any impact on one can affect the other two. And the most impactful way to keep this complex at peak health is through Balanced Breathing. Balanced Breathing simply means breathing the way it should be.

Balanced Breathing may sound very simple. But it is actually not so. The simple reason it is not so is that breathing is simply not a conscious phenomenon. It is an involuntary process in our body. Fortunately for us, nearly every involuntary process in our body can be tweaked by us to an extent. For example, the heartbeat is an involuntary process, but we can change it to an extent, such as raising it through exercise and lowering it by resting.

Balanced Breathing is the way nature intended breathing to be: correct breathing. Unfortunately, the pressures of living of can cause this balance to go awry. Stress, thoughts and emotions change the way we breathe without our realizing it. The result is a dysfunctional autonomic nervous system, which leads to numerous diseases with acid reflux being one of the manifestations. Breathing is directly connected to the Spirit or the intelligence that drives our autonomic nervous system. By correcting breathing, we can tweak our autonomic nervous system to peak health.

So, as you can now see, Balanced Breathing and respiratory health is the key to correcting acid reflux. In the ensuing chapters, you will read about the various ways in which you can achieve Balanced Breathing. Balanced Breathing can be brought on track by improving Lung Capacity through certain breathing exercises. But the best results are achieved when this backed up by proper diet and thought management. So, the various ways to improve Lung Capacity are thus aligned along three axes: Diet (for the Body), simple Breathing Exercises (for the Spirit) and Emotional Management (for the Mind).

Don't forget, the three pillars of the complex are always intertwined, anything done for one also affecting the other two.

In fact, most of the other digestive ailments like IBD (Inflammatory Bowel Disease) can be treated by improving the respiratory health. Several studies have shown a strong correlation between GERD and lung function. Some studies have concluded that GERD causes respiratory issues. But the association of smoking with GERD, and IBD with respiratory illnesses (COPD) have corroborated the connection between respiratory health and digestive troubles that yoga teachers have always alluded to.

Research has also shown that deep breathing exercises significantly decrease the incidence of GERD. In effect, any solution that does not work on the respiratory capabilities and lung function has little chance of curing GERD. Not all people with acid reflux will have COPD. But by raising pulmonary health and capability, acid reflux can certainly be mitigated.

Similarly, a high prevalence of GERD in people with psychiatric diagnosis and in type A people establishes a link between GERD and thought patterns. The respiratory system is thus central to the autonomic nervous system that regulates the involuntary activities of all the other systems like the digestive, excretory and circulatory systems. The association of depression and anxiety in people with COPD only further confirms the nexus between respiratory function and GERD, COPD, IBD and clinical depression. In fact, improving lung functioning can dramatically help with autoimmune diseases like Rheumatoid arthritis.

The summary of all this is that any line of treatment for acid reflux must include all the three MBS aspects for an effective and lasting cure. As most regimens don't, this explains the mystery of acid reflux and why it is normally not tractable to a permanent cure.

# 3 THE MIRACLE OF SMALL MEALS

The incidence of acid reflux disease varies from region to region. The highest levels in many countries could be as high as 30% with the lowest of around 8% in eastern Asians. While there could be various reasons to explain this wide variation in incidence, a quick analysis indicates that lower consumption of sugar, fat and milk could be keeping the incidence of acid reflux low in East Asians.

The typical treatment for acid reflux involves antacids, H2 blockers and PPIs. Antacids contain primarily compounds of aluminium, magnesium or calcium and work by neutralizing the stomach acid. H2 blockers and PPIs work by stopping the secretion of the stomach acid though the mechanisms in both are different.

H2 blockers work by inhibiting histamine at the H2 histamine receptor sites in the parietal cells of the stomach that secrete hydrochloric acid. Ranitidine is the most popular generic drug (as in Zantac) in this category. Proton Pump Inhibitors or PPIs work by stopping the proton pumps in the parietal cells. The proton pumps' normal function is to release the hydrogen ions into the stomach, making the stomach contents acidic. Omeprazole, esomeprazole and rabeprazole are some of the generic drugs in this category.

PPIs have largely overtaken H2 blockers in the treatment of acid reflux due to their increased effectiveness. Your doctor will tell you which medicine is most suitable for you. The aim of this book is to reduce the symptoms of acid reflux through tricks with diet, simple breathing exercises and emotions management. As the symptoms reduce, your doctor will reduce the medication, and gradually you may be able to stop them completely under the doctor's guidance. However, it is very important to consciously watch the symptoms and, in consultation with your doctor, explore every possibility to decrease the dosage, the symptoms permitting. As PPIs usage is reduced, rebound acid formation may happen due to release of excessive gastrin, and in such cases, it is better to treat such acid reflux or occasional acid reflux with antacids or H2 blockers, which are less habit-forming than the PPIs, so as to wean oneself from the dependence-forming PPIs. That's why one should wean off PPIs gradually and not go cold turkey.

Acid reflux is caused by stomach acid backing up into the esophagus due to improper closing of the Lower Esophageal Sphincter (LES), which is like a valve at the entrance to the stomach. The main symptom of acid reflux is heartburn or a burning sensation in the food pipe. Heartburn is most severe sometime after a meal. Other symptoms include sore throat, persistent cough, chest pain, breathing difficulties, sour belching, excessive belching, flatulence, bloating, stomach pain and mouth ulcers.

Ironically, people using medicines for acid reflux may also develop stomach ulcers. Some people with reflux also develop a Geographic Tongue (tongue with "maps"), and others may experience a loss of tooth enamel. The symptoms are quite wide ranging and vary with individuals. Some also experience pain in the left hand and between the shoulder blades. It is not uncommon for people with acid reflux to experience headaches or tightness in the head and redness in the eyes. People with acid reflux are also prone to a racing heart and panic attacks.

The most effective natural method to decrease the symptoms of heartburn and acid reflux is to have small meals. Depending on what the current meal size is, the meal can gradually be decreased by 10% initially to as much as 50%. The guideline here for the meal size is that one should feel very light and comfortable on getting up from a meal. To reinforce this idea: "One should feel just as light on getting up after a meal as before sitting down for it."

Typically, we should eat up to about 60% of our capacity. This is one action that brings about an instant result. Within a couple of hours, the stomach starts easing, the heartburn subsides, the bloating sensation is gone, and you start zipping around with gusto. In a couple of days, the belly gets tucked in, the skin tone improves and a sense of exuberance rises. Small meals reduce the appetite, creating a virtuous circle that puts you on a high. After tasting this newfound sense of high, one no longer feels any regret in giving up on some of their favourite foods.

Initially, it is tough to get up from a small meal. But by telling ourselves that we can eat again, if needed, after a couple of hours, we will get the strength to quit the meal. Even if the total food intake remains the same (though it will eventually go down) due to the increased frequency of the smaller meals, the benefits still remain. This is because a small meal decreases the spikes in blood sugar. Smaller peaks in blood sugar bring in an enormous number of benefits, apart from an improvement in heartburn symptoms, ranging from weight loss, improved skin tone, improvements in blood lipid profile to elimination of body aches and pains. Moreover, smaller peaks in blood sugar levels lower insulin levels, leading to a reduction in hunger.

However, smaller meals are easier said than done. Very soon, old habits start kicking in, and there will be a relapse to past ways. It requires a number of attempts, constant motivation and continual consciousness to make this happen consistently. With a little persistence, small meals decrease hunger levels that eventually lead to lower overall intake of food.

Overall reduction of carbohydrates and sugars significantly decreases acid levels in the stomach over time, and small meals eventually cause this effect. Sugar should be restricted to no more than 4-6 teaspoons a day; the lesser the better, zero being the ideal. The benefits begin to appear almost instantly. Initially, this process may appear tough, but once the benefits are experienced and the realization sets in that there are far greater joys in eating less than in eating more, the motivation to continue comes easily.

In traditional yogic wisdom, food is self-perpetuating. The more you have it, the more you will want it, irrespective of whether your body truly needs it as much or not. Some advocate the complete elimination of carbohydrates, instead of cutting the meal size. This might sometimes be helpful in decreasing acid reflux, but too much of fat or protein (to compensate for the loss of carbohydrates) is never good in the long run and can cause many other health complications. In fact, some people who changed to a higher protein and lower carbohydrate diet had developed acid reflux subsequently.

A drastic change in diet is never a good idea. For many people, changing their diet composition is practically very difficult to sustain, and can cause difficulties to the family and to social life. Moreover, the body does need some carbohydrates. The problem is only when the carbohydrate (and especially sugar) is too high. Instead of increasing protein or fat to substitute for the carbohydrates, it is easier to reduce the meal size or substitute with easily available vegetables. Salads, vegetables and sprouts not only replace the carbohydrates well but also bring in a whole host of health benefits. People who are not used to raw foods should gradually increase the intake of raw vegetables as any sudden diet changes can cause stomach upsets. Interestingly, many people find that fatty food triggers reflux.

There appears to be a complex interplay of multiple factors in acid reflux. While excessive sugars and carbohydrates can worsen reflux, studies have also shown that carbohydrates, fats and sugars under certain conditions (that we shall see later) are the best foods to naturally decrease heartburn symptoms.

Sometimes, stomach ulcers accompany acid reflux. In fact, prolongued use of acid-suppressing drugs increases the chances of getting ulcers. Loss of stomach acid during the medication can lead to increased H. pylori infection in the stomach, and this bacteria increases ulceration in the stomach. It is often seen that H. pylori presence leads to lower incidence of acid reflux, but prolongued usage of acid-suppressing drugs can lead to a peculiar situation of H. pylori presence along with acid reflux. Interestingly, this sharply conflicts with the short-term triple therapy, with PPIs as one component, used in H. pylori eradication protocols. This complex interplay of factors in acid reflux only reflects our limited understanding of the complex mechanics of acid reflux.

If ulcers are persistent, small meals may become difficult initially and binge eating may result, worsening the situation. Spicy and fried food should be avoided when there are ulcers. Small amounts of cheese and healthy fats will help. Honey works great in relieving the gnawing pain of ulcers. Small quantities of sweet food (preferably sweetened by honey, fruits or even brown sugar like muscovado, brown rock sugar or jaggery) at the end of the meal (keep in mind though the incompatible food combinations explained later) will bring in satiety to reduce the cravings caused by ulcers. Even foods sweetened by sugar will help in such situations, bringing relief in the short-term, but sugar will eventually worsen the condition.

However, the trick with all these items is that they should be taken in moderation to get the benefits. When taken in excess, they not only exacerbate acid reflux but also create a host of other problems. In any case, as soon as the ulcers subside, sugar should be cut to stop the acid reflux. Eventually, however, eating small meals at frequent intervals, while cutting sugars, is the best way to cure ulcers too. One has to patiently go through this back and forth process till things stabilize, and stabilize they will with persistence.

Some people claim that acid reflux is due to less acid in the stomach, and consumption of acidic food like apple cider vinegar helps. Others find that eating sour foods increases symptoms of heartburn. The guide in such situations is that if nausea, which goes away on eating something sour, is experienced then there was less acid. Otherwise, predominantly, acid reflux appears to be due to excess stomach acid. In either case, eating too much of sour food in a meal is never advisable. Apple cider vinegar (ACV) or any other natural vinegar like coconut vinegar or citrus fruits should be taken at least half an hour before food. Some people can also experience acid reflux due to physical conditions like hiatal hernia.

Interestingly, intensive weight training or physical exercise appears to trigger reflux. Many bodybuilders and an estimated 50% of pregnant women suffer from reflux. This could be an indication that acid reflux may not always be due to high or low stomach acid but that the bigger culprit could also be a poorly-functioning LES or abnormal pressure in the stomach or on the LES.

Sour foods such as diluted apple cider vinegar (ACV) or citrus fruits or sour fruit juices should always be taken on an empty stomach. Taken 30-60 minutes before a meal, they do not cause any discomfort. On the other hand, having them along with a meal is a sure recipe for heartburn. In particular, a spoon of ACV in a glass of water works wonders for many people with heartburn. Incidentally, per yoga teachers, fruit should always be eaten alone and never mixed with other food to get the maximum benefits. Citrus fruits, as long as they are not too sour, should definitely be eaten on an empty stomach by people with acid reflux. Then they do not cause any discomfort. On the other hand, they are considered to be alkalinizing in nature and will eventually reduce acid reflux.

However, vinegar, like lime juice, should be taken highly diluted to avoid its corrosive effect on teeth enamel and lining of the esophagus. Ginger, anise seeds, fennel seeds, cinnamon etc. do help in improving digestive health (again, the caution here is to use them in moderation as their excess consumption can cause other problems; criteria for spices usage follows soon), but they do not help in very severe acid reflux. PPIs for a short duration are still the best choice for treating severe acid reflux (and it is important to quickly bring down the symptoms of heartburn to prevent the erosion of the esophagus and other complications), but with meal size reduction PPIs can be dropped soon or their dosage can easily be reduced.

Like ACV, another very good item that can lead to an overall improvement in acid reflux is warm lime-honey water. A glass of limewater mixed with a spoon of honey taken on an empty stomach can steadily ease many of the stomach discomforts. It is particularly helpful in easing bloating and intestinal pain. Make sure that the limewater is dilute enough to be pleasantly or mildly sour. The honey should be added when the water is warm and not hot. Honey loses its benefits when added to hot water (and becomes poison per yoga teachers). And rinse your mouth after drinking the limewater so that any deleterious effects on teeth enamel are washed out.

Food combinations are another important aspect for the long-term treatment of acid reflux. The following combinations are considered bad: protein-starch, protein-sour food, mixed starches, mixed proteins, starch-sugar, fat-sugar, starch-acid, protein-fat and protein-sugar. The good combinations are starch-fats, fats-sour foods and sugar-sour foods. So, bread and meat are a bad food combination, as also meat and orange juice or bread and jam. On the other hand, sweet citrus fruits, even soft drinks like colas (due to the good sugar-sour combination, though the high sugar is a negative) or bread-butter digest easily.

Green leafy vegetables and non-starchy vegetables are a good choice with any kind of food. So, we can see that for people with a sudden attack of heartburn a good food to eat is salads with olive oil and small quantities of lemon juice or vinegar. If you want to eat cereals or grains with this, avoid the lemon and vinegar. Another good combination is bread-butter with vegetables.

But if you have to eat meat, take it with non-starchy vegetables without fatty dressings (sprinkling salt or spices on the vegetables can help with the taste). Similarly, sweet citrus fruits when taken alone digest well and keep stomach acid low (the acid in the fruit suppresses the stomach acidity; in addition, due to their alkaline ash, citrus fruit help in the eventual reduction of stomach acid). However, when orange juice or a soft drink is taken with a meal containing protein or starch, the result can be bloating (due to the bad sugar-protein or sugar-starch combinations).

Some people find that fatty food triggers reflux. This may be due to bad combinations of fatty food. On the other hand, if starch-fat is eaten, there will very likely be an improvement in heartburn.

Milk should ideally be taken alone. At best, it can be combined with vegetables and cereals. Natural yoghurt and fruits are also a good combination. Milk and yoghurt are best taken moderately and that too diluted with equal parts of water. Thick milk is hard to digest. Thick milk or yoghurt with sugar can easily trigger reflux. In contrast, diluted yoghurt, salted or sweetened, can soothe heartburn.

Food combinations can work differently with different people. People with a robust digestive system may be more tolerant to bad food combinations. For the more sensitive others, respecting the rules of good food combination always helps. However, due to the constraints of modern life, it may not be possible to always adhere to these rules. In such cases, small meals may nullify the deleterious effects of any bad combination.

Obsessing unnecessarily over such matters is actually counter-productive, because as we shall see later mental and emotional disharmony is more harmful than diet itself. It is enough if the rules are practised as much as is practically possible. When combined with the other changes that we shall see later, the results will be good enough. Where one has to be extra careful is where the meal has multiple incompatible combinations.

To get an idea of how ideal meals look like, a breakfast could consist of only fruit with or without diluted yoghurt or protein with vegetables. Lunch or supper could be salads and fat with a little vinegar or lime juice, or cereals with fat and vegetables. However, if your lifestyle does not permit such meals, you can have some protein, limited carbohydrates with a little fat. Avoid sour foods and sugars with such a meal. Cereals and lentils in moderation could also be eaten together. For people with acid reflux, and particularly those also with ulcers, eating a light meal of starch with vegetables and washing it down with a small quantity of sweetened diluted yogurt at the end can be very soothing.

People with acid reflux should avoid desserts, especially when the symptoms are manifest. For those unable to resist a sweet dish during a meal, have it at the end of a meal of starches and vegetables (with low protein and low fat). Avoid desserts with high sugar, high fat and high starches (such as cakes with a lot of icing) and choose instead either concentrated sugar types such as candies or ones with less sugar or less starch or less fat and more fruit or vegetable (such as pumpkin) or with more chocolate. Eating sugar with starch (like in bread and jam or cakes with plenty of icing) at the same time causes the enzyme ptyalin, necessary for the digestion of starch, to stay away from the saliva. But if you can't avoid such a dessert, then just have a smaller helping.

Sucking on a small candy at the end of a starchy meal helps in the easy digestion of the starch by decreasing the stomach acid, but don't do this if you've had plenty of protein because protein needs stomach acid to get digested. However, remember eating too much sugar eventually raises the stomach acid.

If all these sound a bit complex, just follow this rule of thumb to instantly mitigate heartburn: eat a simple, small meal with as few varied items (minimalist) as you can. Be more careful when the symptoms of reflux are strong, and pamper yourself a little when the symptoms are down.

Good practices play a very important role in maintaining digestive health that will eventually reduce acid reflux. Bananas are best eaten alone and slightly raw. Plantains (raw bananas cooked as vegetables) are very good for high acid stomachs because they not only go well with starches and form a protective coating in the stomach lining but also have a low glycemic index (GI) compared to ripe bananas. Low GI foods are definitely a plus for acid reflux.

Avoid taking liquids or water half an hour before a meal and for two hours after it. This will keep the stomach light, facilitate good digestion and keep the glycemic index of the meal lower. This is a particularly effective solution for those experiencing bloating or pain shortly after a meal. Eat slowly and mindfully to stem the urge to drink water.

It is a good practice to finish the night meal at least two hours before going to bed. A well-digested and light meal makes sleep very refreshing, and good sleep is very important for mitigating acid reflux. Drinking a small glass of warm milk diluted with equal parts of water at bedtime helps in relaxing and sleeping well. We should avoid any mentally or physically strenuous work after supper. In fact, we should just relax, spend time with family, do some light reading or take a light stroll before winding up another blessed day. Avoid exposure to high-voltage excitement on TV and intense reading on the PC or mobile as they disturb restful sleep.

Watching engrossing programmes on TV while eating is quite bad for the stomach because the mind and body are raised to a high, and adequate blood flow to the stomach is not available. After lunch, it is necessary to relax for 15 minutes before taking up any kind of strenuous work. But go for a stroll (not brisk walking though) after supper.

People suffering from acid reflux should work on all these areas to get a lasting cure. The best part of doing all this is that these practices not only cure the acid reflux, but they also bestow us with high energy, a feeling of lightness, an overall improvement in fitness and health and reduce stress. The domino effect will also be visible in happier and more loving relationships.

Another important lifestyle requirement is having a regulated life. The body has its own biological clock, and respecting this clock does a great deal for health. This includes eating and sleeping, as far as possible, at regular timings. Waking up early between 4:30 am and 6 am not only increases our chances to complete our daily physical exercises, but they make our days more productive and satisfying. This is because, in the circadian rhythm that our bodies follow, our bodies are so tuned that waking up in this period bestows us with peak physical capabilities and high mental faculties. Going by the same circadian rhythm, we should aim to sleep between 9:30 pm and 11 pm.

Exercise, especially Yoga, is best done on any empty stomach. Traditional wisdom says that our breakfast should be light, lunch heavier and dinner light again. Fruits should be taken on an empty stomach but preferably before 6 pm. Pulpy fruits, especially, like papaya and guava are best eaten before sunset, to avoid poor digestion and phlegm formation. Yoghurt should be avoided in the night.

Gut health and gut flora are increasingly being recognized for their impact on good digestion. Fermented vegetables and natural yoghurt with live culture are, therefore, a great way to improve digestion and absorption. However, the fermentation should be controlled (by adding smaller quantities of starter culture and refrigerating early) as too sour foods should always be avoided. Ideally, foods should not be too salty, too sweet, too sour or too pungent. Fresh, freshly prepared, and tasty yet mild foods not only keep the stomach cool but also the mind calm.

In traditional wisdom, water has a tremendous memory. It carries the thoughts, feelings and emotions of the people and places around it. So, food cooked by family members with love and care does a great deal for our own mental and physical health. Of course in modern life, this is not always possible, but one should try as much as possible to eat home-cooked food. If you believe in God that's great because traditional wisdom says that a prayer is picked by the water in our food and blesses us with physical health and mental harmony.

When we are constrained to eat outside foods, we can at least try and avoid food processed at very high temperatures, with chemicals, preservatives and binders, with trans fats, too much sodium etc. Raw food or food cooked not earlier than three hours before eating are the best. Steamed food is the ideal cooked food, while baked and fried foods, which are subjected to high temperatures are best eaten minimum. Olive oil for salads, coconut oil for cooking and clarified butter (the Indian variety is ghee) are good fats. Ghee is an excellent remedy for ulcers, but like all fats should be eaten moderately. Needless to add, smoking and alcohol should be restricted as much as possible.

Nightshade vegetables like tomatoes, potatoes, peppers and eggplants are best avoided in the regimen for acid reflux. Tomatoes are ideally eaten cooked with the seeds removed. Cucumbers should be eaten with seeds removed. The foods that are most beneficial in the treatment of acid reflux are squashes, in particular ash gourd (also known as winter melons) and bottle gourd (also known as calabash). They are best taken raw, juiced or as salads. They are not only very effective in calming the stomach but also the mind, making our days energetic and nights restful.

In Ayurveda, some foods are heating in their internal effect, while others are cooling. This has nothing to do with their temperatures though. Food like ginger and most spices are heating in their internal effect on the body. On the other hand, spices like turmeric, coriander seeds, fennel and cumin are cooling. For people with reflux, it is very important to avoid heating foods and choose cooling foods. So, even though ginger and cinnamon generally aid in digestion, they are best avoided during severe reflux. On the other hand, drinking a glass of diluted yoghurt with a little salt and powdered cumin seeds an hour before a meal can be very helpful. Similarly, drinking warm milk spiced with a little turmeric powder at bedtime can ease heartburn. Again, chewing on a mixture of fennel and roasted coriander seeds after meals is very helpful.

# 4 THE VITAL AIR

As we have seen earlier, all the subconscious or involuntary activities are interconnected, and a disturbance in one eventually affects many other systems. Through small meals, we can actually enhance our pulmonary capability. In fact, many benefits of yoga become available through moderation in eating. Further, without moderation in eating, no yoga can bestow full benefits.

Breathing exercises are another way of maintaining peak respiratory health, which, in turn, drives the digestive system. A healthy digestive system, in turn, maintains the other systems in peak health. Apart from people with acid reflux, all those suffering from other digestive ailments such as IBD, skin ailments, breathing ailments, rheumatoid arthritis and psychiatric issues will hugely benefit from this chapter.

Balanced Breathing is the way breathing ought to be. Without getting into too many technicalities, it will be interesting to note that carbon dioxide or $CO_2$ in our blood is an important parameter of our health. While the importance of good oxygen supply is well known, the importance of $CO_2$ level in blood is not widely understood. Correct $CO_2$ levels help in maintaining blood pH, oxygen absorption at the cellular level and in the smooth functioning of the digestive tract. On the other hand, rapid and shallow breathing decrease $CO_2$ in the blood and alter body chemistry that in the long-term causes diseases.

In balanced breathing, breathing is slow and deeper, with exhalation twice as long as inhalation. This ensures optimal blood

CO2 levels, and good availability and absorption of oxygen at the cellular level. This balance is often disturbed by wrong food habits and stress. The good news is that there are breathing exercises designed to help get our breathing back in balance naturally. They are very effective, especially when backed by changes in diet and by the way we think.

Modern research has also shown that people who practice deep breathing achieve significant reduction in the symptoms of acid reflux. Studies have also shown that breathing exercises achieve vagal nerve stimulation and better heart rate variability, both of which help us to manage stress better. The entire mechanics by which Balanced Breathing and breathing exercises improve our body chemistry are not fully known, but there is enough evidence to demonstrate a clear correlation between correct breathing and health.

Ancient yogis had an uncanny understanding of the relationship between breathing and body chemistry. They had developed a highly advanced science of breathing called Pranayama. While highly beneficial, some of these breathing exercises can be quite complex and if not practiced correctly under strict the guidance of a guru can cause a lot of harm. The complex ones require a certain lifestyle or regimen as a precondition. Practising them without that lifestyle adjustment or in an incorrect way can lead to problems. However, there are some breathing exercises in Pranayama that are safe, particularly those that do not involve the prolongued holding of breath. These exercises are safe for anyone to do, including all of us in the modern lifestyle. Of them, in particular, **Anuloma Viloma** or the single nostril breathing is very effective for the health of the autonomic nervous system, and eventually for the treatment of acid reflux.

Practice of Anuloma Viloma not only increases the lung capacities and pulmonary health but also helps in many incurable diseases. People with acid reflux should practice this breathing exercise regularly. Here is the method for practicing it:

1. Sit cross-legged on a mat with the back as straight as possible. A mat is mandated during yoga to avoid transfer of body currents to the ground.
2. The entire back, neck and head should be absolutely straight. Again, a straight spine is very essential for the proper flow of

certain energies through the spine.

3.  Adjust the legs so that the maximum part of the buttocks, thighs and the knees are in contact with the ground. This is the Sukhasana posture. The hands should rest on the knees with the palms facing upwards. Every aspect of the posture is so designed that long spells of sitting create minimal strain. To illustrate, as the maximum load is transferred to the buttocks and thighs, there is less stress on the lower back. With hands outstretched and palms facing upwards, there is additional support for the torso, leading to a relaxed posture.

4.  Fold the index and middle fingers of the right hand while keeping the other fingers straight. With the elbow down, gently close the right nostril with the thumb finger, and breathe in deeply through the left nostril. Focus the mind on the lungs, and breathe deeply so that you can feel the lungs expanding gently like a balloon.

5.  Now close the left nostril with the pinky and ring fingers, and breathe out slowly through the right nostril. Then breathe in deeply through the right nostril and close the right nostril with the thumb. Breathe out slowly through the left nostril by releasing the pinky and little fingers. Repeat the cycle.

6.  The ingenuity of the finger configuration can be realized when even after 15 minutes of this breathing the right hand or shoulder does not tire.

7.  Start with a few rounds initially, and gradually increase to 9 rounds every day. The time for breathing in and out should be the same. Initially, this may be about 2 seconds, and one can soon reach 6 seconds.

8.  There should be no holding of breath between breathing in and out. The entire exercise should be done effortlessly, and there should be no exertion or forcing of oneself at any point. The duration of each round should gradually be raised as the lung capacity increases. Your body is your best guide and if you observe any strain, stop and start again when you are more comfortable.

9.  Gradually, the ratio of inhalation to exhalation should be increased to 1: 2. Research has confirmed that slow or extended exhalation raised the benefits of breathing exercises.

Two other exercises **Brahmari** and **Omkar** are also very effective in increasing pulmonary health for the common person (if you are under the guidance of a yoga guru, you can practise the more advanced techniques, but the simple exercises specified here are adequate for normal purposes).

In Brahmari, sitting in the Sukhasana posture, plug the ears with the thumbs, with the index fingers resting on the forehead just above the eyebrow and the other three fingers covering the eyeball snugly (see illustrations at the end of the chapter). Take a deep breath (fill the lungs) through both the nostrils, and release it gradually while making a humming sound at the throat. Feel the vibration in the face during the hum.

In Omkar, the hands are resting on the knees again, with palms facing upwards. The breathing-in is the same as in Brahmari, but while breathing out say 'Om' slowly to last the duration of the exhalation. The last 30% of the Om should be with the lips closed (so as to hum 'mmmm').

Both these exercises can be done for three to five rounds. Here the restriction to 3-5 rounds is because the breathing out is restrained (and any holding of breath requires a certain regimen to be followed under the guidance of a guru) due to the humming activity. For expert yogis, whose bodies are extremely fit and who have achieved peak lung capabilities whilst following many other lifestyle regulations, the number of rounds and duration of each round can be much higher. For us, the normal folks, the durations specified here are adequate for our purposes and do not carry the risk of overstrain.

Brahmari and Omkar may appear very simple, and one may even wonder if such simple exercises could really be efficacious. It is to be noted that in these two exercises, it is possible to reduce respiratory rate from the usual 12-15 per minute to just 2-3 respirations per minute. The prolongued exhalation stimulates vagal tone and raises respiratory sinus arrhythmia (RSA), which is the natural heart rate variation during each breathing cycle. A higher heart rate variability is desired for good heart health. In yoga, certain sound frequencies (as in these two exercises) are considered to generate neurological benefits. Brahmari and Omkar are thus very effective in the treatment of acid reflux.

Studies have shown that people who exercise have better pulmonary health, as determined in the Pulmonary Function Test

(PFT), than others. But people who practise yoga are found to be even better, especially in achieving peak expiration flow rates. The breathing exercises in yoga increase lung capacity (decrease of intrapulmonary shunt and consequent dead space reduction) and reduce bronchial airway resistance.

At the end, continuing in the Sukhasana posture, breathe in deeply and breathe out slowly. In deep breathing-in, the lungs expand and the stomach goes out. In breathing out, the stomach goes in as the lungs contract. This **Deep Breathing** can be done for 10-20 minutes. Those constrained by time, other reasons or by a recent surgery for ears, nose or throat can choose to do only Deep Breathing, once or twice a day, as part of the breathing regimen to cure acid reflux. Deep Breathing for 3 rounds can be done whenever required, but for longer durations, one should avoid the first couple of hours after a meal. In Deep Breathing too, one can gradually increase the inhalation to exhalation ratio to 1:2 to maximize the benefits.

Another important breathing exercise (Pranayama) for decreasing bronchial airway resistance is the **Bhastrika**. For doing this, kneel down and sit on legs, buttocks resting on the feet with the toes pointing backwards and the bridge of the foot touching the ground. The back, neck and head should be ramrod straight and in a straight line. This is the Vajrasana posture. With the fists closed and thumbs on top, keep the fists ahead of the shoulders, elbows level with the shoulders. The fists should face each other.

Inhaling forcefully, simultaneously open both hands, while opening the fists with outstretched fingers fully wide and in line with the shoulders, with speed and force (the action resembles opening out a jacket). Then, closing the fists, bring the hands to the original position (action like wearing a jacket on) till the fists are ahead of the shoulders while exhaling forcefully. To reiterate, open the hands wide while forcefully inhaling, and close the hands while forcefully exhaling.

Repeat the cycle 18 times. After a break, repeat another round of 18 cycles. A total of three such rounds can be practised.

Remember that when a certain level of proficiency in these breathing exercises is attained, while breathing in the chest expands and the stomach goes out. While breathing out, the chest falls in and the stomach goes in. In the rhythmic and fast breathing in and out during Bhastrika, the stomach keeps rhythmically going out and in.

To attain a very effective breathe-out, it is good to slightly and consciously tuck the stomach in.

The ingenuity of the Vajarasana posture for this exercise is that the body is extremely stable in the forceful breathing in and out. The same stability cannot be attained in, say, Sukhasana posture.

Bhastrika can be rather strenuous for people with poor pulmonary capacity. It is better to start with Anuloma Viloma, Brahmari, Omkar and Deep Breathing for a few days. When the improvements in lung capacity are significantly perceptible, Bhastrika should be attempted. In this case, the correct sequence is Bhastrika, Anuloma Viloma, Brahmari, Omkar and Deep Breathing.

Do not eat or drink anything for a minimum of 10 minutes after completing the breathing exercises. For maximum effectiveness, the exercises should be done with eyes closed and in mindfulness. Along with these breathing exercises, doing other physical exercises like the Yoga postures or aerobic exercises like walking will help in accelerating the stopping of all acid reflux. Pregnant women and people with uncontrolled blood pressure or heart disease should not attempt Bhastrika.

Posture is a very important aspect of respiratory capability. People who sit for long hours, especially, tend to have a decreased lung capacity. Sitting straight will better maintain respiratory capability. People with acid reflux will, therefore, have to take care to prevent slouching while sitting, standing or while lounging in the bed or the sofa.

Food containing magnesium is proven to be good for respiratory health. Green leafy vegetables, nuts, pumpkin and sesame seeds (which are normally easily available) are rich in magnesium. Sesame seeds are also a good source of selenium, another mineral that greatly benefits respiratory health. Even sesame oil has been proven to be effective in improving respiratory health. Needless to write, all nuts, seeds and oils need to be taken in moderation. As sesame seeds are heating in nature, people with reflux should certainly exercise moderation in eating them and particulary avoid them when heartburn is severe.

In yoga, the spinal cord occupies a place of importance in the functioning of the autonomic nervous system (ANS). Yoga recommends daily exercises for the spine and for spinal flexibility. The various yoga asanas or postures are designed to achieve this spinal health. So, if you are not practicing any Yoga postures, make sure you keep the spine supple and strong through regular forward and backward bending and twisting exercises, for the proper functioning of the ANS. Not surprisingly, chiropractors, who work on musculoskeletal systems, especially the spine, to correct physical ailments, have been able to claim some successes in the treatment of acid reflux by working on the spine and posture.

It will now be easy to understand why people with acid reflux will have to give up smoking, which significantly decreases the lung capacity and function. As the pulmonary capabilities improve and increase, the digestive system may get completely normalized. At that juncture, it will be possible to eat without restraint and still avoid acid reflux. But my guess is most people still won't break their regimen, even if they can, because the intoxication that stems from the health benefits that come from it will make it addictive. Besides, yoga claims, eating moderately brings a heavenly bliss in the body.

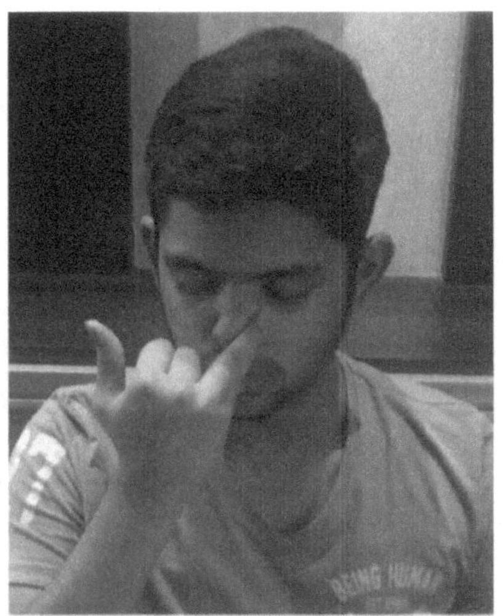

**Breathing through the right nostril
in Anuloma Viloma**

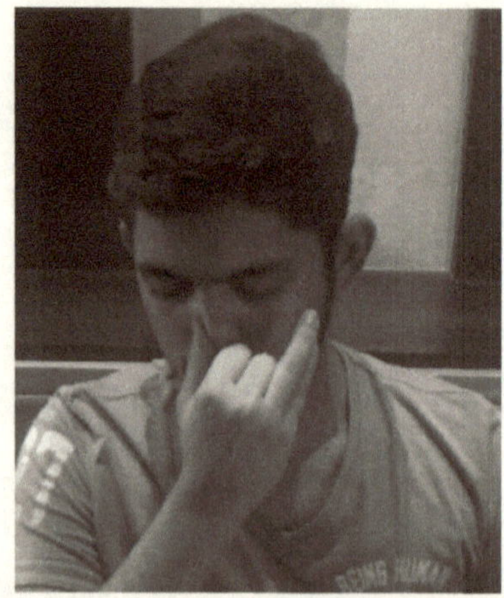

**Breathing through the left nostril
in Anuloma Viloma**

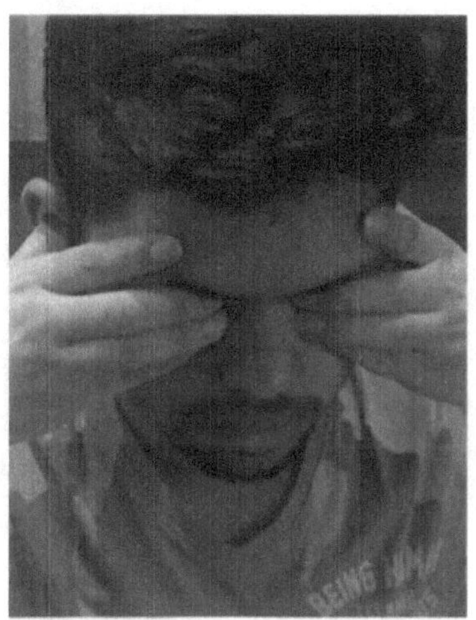

**Ears plugged and eyes covered in
Brahmari**

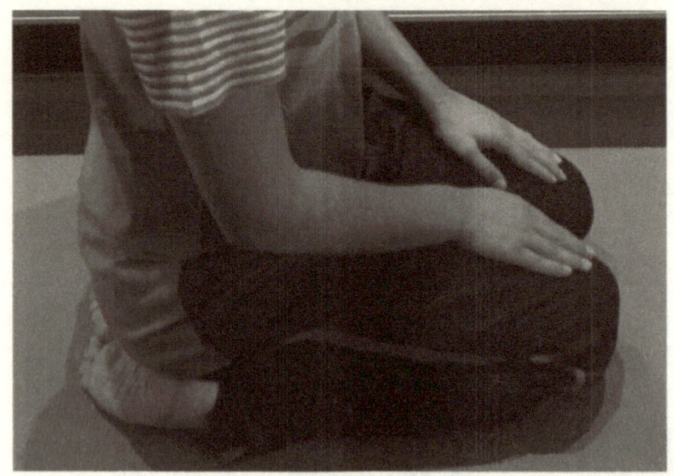

**Sitting in Vajrasana**

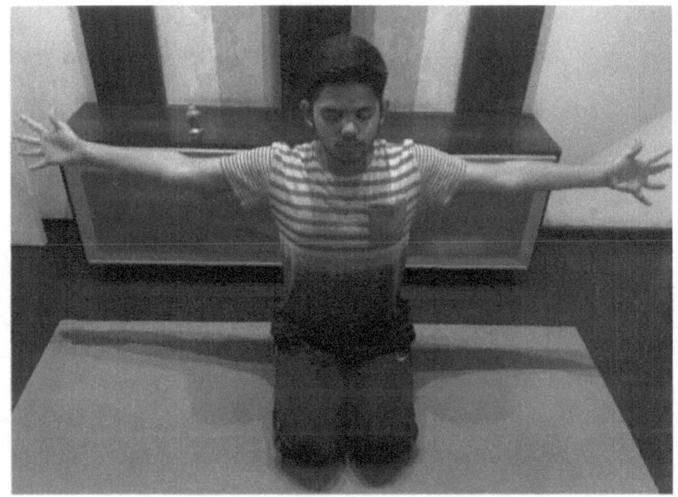

**Forceful breathe-in in Bhastrika
with Vajrasana position**

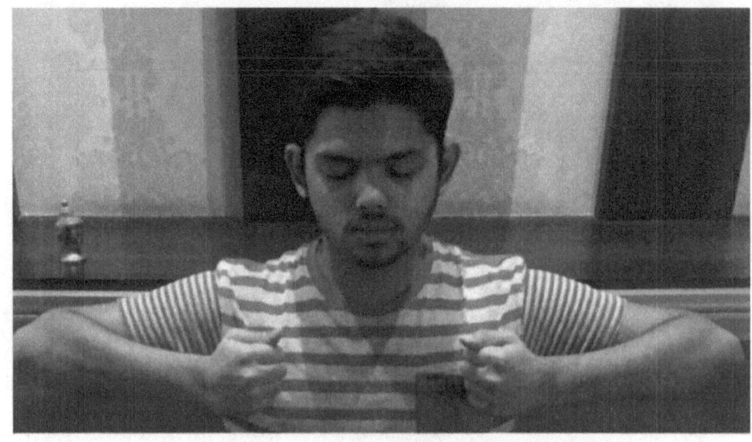

**Forceful breathe-out in Bhastrika
with Vajrasana position**

# 5 SHIFTING FROM 'TAKE' TO 'SERVICE'

In Yoga, the mind plays a very important role in the functioning of the autonomic nervous system. Our thoughts and emotions can make our breathing go awry. So, any plan to cure acid reflux will doubtless involve working on the mental aspects. When diet, breathing, the spine and the mind are worked on simultaneously, acid reflux becomes amenable to control. In most regimes for acid reflux, the emphasis is on diet with exercise and stress reduction thrown in as general health moves that will facilitate the cure. But breathing and emotions management (which is a step beyond stress management) are not just adjuncts to diet control but independent elements in the regimen for the cure of acid reflux.

A question that you might want to ask at this stage may be that when breathing exercises can bring breathing back on the track of balance, is it still necessary to work on the mind to ensure Balanced Breathing? Yoga says that we need to watch our breath constantly, twenty-four hours a day, three hundred and sixty-five days a year. No fix will work effectively if it is not backed up by the right lifestyle. Yoga's benefits rise manifold when there is moderation in eating and drinking, and there is restraint in thinking and doing.

This may sound depressing to the epicureans and the gastronomes. But ask all those around you who eat moderately. The joy of blissful energy and health that comes in the wake of moderate eating and from a positive living is not only intoxicating but also addictive. Once you taste it, other tastes will no longer have their stranglehold on you.

While studies have shown that stress and type A personalities are predisposing factors for developing acid reflux, some people who are apparently not subjected to stressful conditions are also diagnosed with acid reflux. The explanation in such cases could be that some fears might be lurking in their subconscious mind. This might sound like a paradox because typically people with fears (especially fear of failure) are paralyzed by fears and are quite unlike the type A personalities. Actually, in this case, and this where it becomes similar to the type As, fears subconsciously work in an opposite form: generating restlessness and hurry for gain. This hurry for gain is overtly manifest in type As while it remains latent in the people with a strong sense of fears.

This restlessness is frequently manifest in people with acid reflux and even when it is not manifest too it remains in the mind like a constant background music, wrecking havoc on the ANS.

Personality types are hard to change. But the ancient yogis had devised certain emotional exercises by which inherent tendencies and personality traits can be overcome. These exercises can be done by anyone at anytime. Actually, they should be practised at all times. They may sound old-fashioned at first, but they are extremely powerful.

Foremost amongst these exercises is the one involving giving up of anger. Surprising as it may sound, anger actually leads to fear. And fear, in turn, feeds anger. It is not possible to give up anger without a change in our beliefs. Keeping a reasonable ceiling on our wants is a very important step in this process. It is good to have a good life, but it is very important that the mind is not hankering after new things all the time. Such tendencies should be curbed beyond a reasonable point. Else, the unrest in the mind subconsciously creates fear and anger.

Those living life in the fast lane, don't get depressed by this. By all means, do enjoy the goodies if you have them or if you have to. Continue to be ambitious. Nothing wrong in aiming high. Plan what you want, and work out what you have to do. Just make sure that your mind is not constantly hankering after them. Balanced breathing will also help you to disassociate your mind easily from compulsive thought-trains.

The yogis had recommended compassion to all as an antidote to physical ills. Love and compassion directly impact the autonomic nervous system. They release oxytocin, which dissolves fear and anger. Compassion is not a subconscious concept that lies inactively in the background of our awareness. It is an intensely active emotion that should throb in us all the time. It should throb in us when we are with family, with friends and even with our enemies. Even though this is very difficult, it should throb in us even when we are tense or angry.

For the average person, it is difficult to be compassionate in the mould of, say, the Dalai Lama. But with awareness and constant practice, definite progress can be made. And every progress made towards a compassionate nature is a certain guarantee for more health, better relationships and happiness. So, start today!

Feelings of vindictiveness and revenge are highly corrosive and leave their toxic footprints on the autonomic nervous system. The power of love can be realized in one simple experiment. Whenever you feel disturbed and your emotions refuse to calm down, try looking at everything and everyone around with intense feelings of love and compassion. Very soon, you will notice the disturbance fading away and a weight being lifted off your chest. The tension or anger will just melt away.

Fear of social stigma can be overcome by controlling thoughts about social respect and standing. Social standing is actually meaningless because public memory is always short-lived. Most people ignore you when you are not needed, and come back to you when they think they need you. Nearly everyone who lives long enough experiences a down after a period of high and can vouch for this phenomenon. Social standing is only skin-deep and is a reflection of our own self-confidence.

So, becoming comfortable with criticism, by learning to laugh at ourselves and by not taking ourselves too seriously, we can gradually lose the fear of social stigma. Love is the best antidote to all fears. When the heart is filled with compassion, even the fear of social stigma dissolves away. The freedom that comes when this is fear is gone is indescribable; it has only to be experienced.

The yogis had stated that emotions are cyclical in their nature, rising and falling like the ocean waves with no apparent rhyme or reason. In particular, anger and irritation come without a warning, do the damage externally and internally and disappear to come again uninvited. Curbing our possessiveness on situations, events, objects and people and their behaviour arrests these waves. Acceptance of outcomes keeps us cool and composed. If every positive outcome is a reason for celebration, then every negative outcome is an opportunity waiting to be explored. Yet, we should not get elated on success because then we will have the equanimity to stay cool during failures.

Many outstanding people rose to extraordinary heights of achievement by braving through negative outcomes. That's why the yogis had always emphasized that our focus should be on the process, the work or the effort and not on the result or outcome. Obsessing over results actually decreases our efficiency, the quality of our output and generates toxic behaviour that eventually eats into the vitals of the autonomic nervous system. Even obsessing over the right food is not advised. Eating the best of whatever is available is adequate. This is because the real benefits of food are not so much in its nutrients as in their absorption by the digestive system. A peaceful and compassionate person eating simple or ordinary food moderately can absorb more nutrients or all the needed nutrients into the body than a person with a taxed mind eating highly nutritious food.

Being cool does not tantamount to a loss of competitive spirit. In fact, the yogis had advocated intense work and an active life as essential for emotional development, which ultimately leads to peak health, fulfillment in relationships and high productivity. (Blessed are the ones who have to struggle because they have the opportunities to outgrow their fears and grow emotionally, unlike the ones who have it all easy.) Only, instead of setting goals on results, they advocated setting goals on the process, i.e., perfecting the process.

Jealousy has no place in such a scheme because it is extremely damaging to the autonomic nervous system. Jealousy has no place because being on top is not the only dimension to life. There are so many other beautiful aspects to life apart from wealth, position, power and fame, which often have a limited shelf life. In fact, if anger, too many wants and cravings, jealousy and hurry for gain are given up, fear and worrying for safety and security will lose their grip on us. Oxytocin in us will rise and, the yogis stated, the internal bliss (arising from the Spirit) in us will come to the fore, giving us a sense of joy that nothing else can match.

When internal bliss is experienced, everything else becomes secondary including such things as who is right and who is wrong, and who won and who lost. Cravings, thoughts of ownership and personal dominance lead to anxiety. By keeping them at reasonable levels, not only do we remain healthier and happier, but also we are more likely to sustain ourselves in the long run. This calls for ready acceptance of situations, adjustment and acceptance of people's behaviour. The chances are that with peak physical health and mental capabilities attained through right diet, spine exercises and breathing techniques, and emotional mastery, our productivity and creativity may touch so high as to put us in a realm of our own.

By controlling thoughts about food, we can moderate our hunger. When we consciously eat moderately, we experience a variant of the inner bliss. When the source of this bliss is understood, food will no longer retain its vice-like grip on us. We will willingly cut down on food to keep experiencing this bliss and the numerous health and emotional benefits that follow.

We tend to be unhappy or restless or plain dissatisfied with our present because of the wrong perception that the best is yet to come. Actually, say the yogis, the best in life is not an outcome of our life situation but actually is the process of enjoying everything that we do with awareness and mindfulness. Everything else is secondary.

Spiritual guru Jaggi Vasudev says that when he was young he would be lost in such seemingly stupid things as watching a leaf for hours together. But that process opened new vistas of wisdom and made him what he is. So, if you are not yet in your dream job, enjoy every job that you do or have to do. Even doing menial jobs or household chores can be a source of great joy when done with mindfulness and wholeheartedly. In fact, I would recommend some kind of housekeeping, gardening or service work every week as tonic for the spirit. Finding beauty in small things and discovering the magic of life in day-to-day activities is a journey that can best be only experienced.

One need not be the best or have the best to be happy. Doing one's best in every situation is what gives life meaning and deep fulfillment. By drilling this axiom deep down to our DNA, fear will lose its power on us. And acid will stay right where it should be: down inside the stomach, instead of backing up into the esophagus.

Anything that we do, however simple or mundane it may be, has the capacity to give us a high. The high always comes when we do anything with complete involvement; when our mind and action are both focussed on the same thing. When the two are in disharmony, stress arises. And when they are in harmony, there is high oxytocin, serotonin and endorphins, leading to a joyous state. If we understand this secret, life becomes a series of joys even without being in a beach resort at an exotic location or on a luxury liner.

A two-minute analysis will reveal that the only thing over which we truly have control is how we act and react. The rest everything is more an accident than due to our effort. Yet, when we put in our best, things do seem to fall in place. But every experience, good and bad, has to be welcomed. Because life is never perfect nor will it ever be. People have learnt more from failures than from successes.

Here is a simple exercise for the emotions that requires just 3 minutes everyday. Often, our minds become powerless when there is a surge in body chemistry. In effect, we become slaves of the chemicals that surge in our bloodstream. This exercise helps us retain control over ourselves and stem those chemical surges.

1. Sit cross-legged (in Sukhasana, preferably on a mat and avoiding direct contact with the ground) with the spine straight in line with the neck and the head (very important).
2. Keep your eyes closed throughout the session. Imagine a transparent bubble or sphere all around you, filled with gentle creamy-white light.
3. The heart is the seat of all emotions. So bring your attention to your heart and gently focus it there.
4. Now fill your heart with the following three feelings.
5. **Love for all**. Let a ball of soothing and yet luminous pink light fill and surround your heart. It fills your heart with love for everyone and everything around you. Realize that everyone and everything is here to play their own role and for a purpose. Let your attention swim in that ball of light, moving into the centre of your heart and sometimes out of that ball into the outer creamy-white bubble. Affirmations are autosuggestions that work powerfully at a neurological level. So, affirm: "Love all, help all. I am always eager to help all." Move your attention between the outer bubble, the inner ball and the affirmation.
6. **Bliss or pure joy**. Then allow the ball of light around your heart to change its colour to a bright but soothing, pure

white. It then fills your heart with unadulterated joy and fulfillment that stays throughout the day and the night. Let your attention swim in that ball of light, moving into the centre of your heart and sometimes out of that ball into the outer creamy-white bubble. Repeat the affirmation: "In the midst of everything I do, I am filled with constant joy and bliss". Move your attention between the outer bubble, the inner ball and the affirmation.

7. **Acceptance or surrender to a higher purpose**. Allow the ball of light to now change its colour to a bright, luminous green. Allow it to fill your heart with a surrender to life, to a higher purpose, where your role is only to do your best. Sparks of white light emerge from the centre of your heart and slowly radiate into the inner ball. At the same time, sparks of brilliant green light are flying slowly all over in the outer bubble of creamy-white light. Repeat the affirmation: "I am always doing my best, and there is only so much I can do. I receive all life events and situations with peaceful acceptance." Allow your attention to drift between the inner ball with its white sparks, the outer bubble with its green sparks, and the affirmation.

8. Practise this exercise for whatever duration you are comfortable with. Even 3 5 minutes is good enough. Do it once or twice a day, or whenever you want to. The longer and the more you do, the better is the impact.

This exercise may seem deceivingly simple but it is a powerful visualization technique, which impacts at a neurological level. Colours have their own effect on our mind and, when used judiciously, can supplement our efforts. The above simple exercise performed regularly over time will have a therapeutic effect, cleansing our heart of all the negativity accumulated over years and bestowing us with the power to tone down and fine-tune our body chemistry.

Let us look at the above three feelings in a bit more detail to understand how they work.

- Now, emotions management begins with anger management. Without mastering anger, it is very difficult to master other emotions. Anger leads to emotional reasoning rather than logical reasoning, causing innocent things to be misinterpreted, which again triggers anger.

- One of the triggers for anger is real or perceived ill treatment or a wrongdoing by someone. A feeling of love for all diminishes the impact that arises due to ill treatment at the hands of or a wrongdoing by another.
- Blissful feelings raise us from a low frustration point (a predisposition for anger) to a high endurance level, cushioning us from the blows of life.
- An inability to deal with problems is another reason for anger. When there is an acceptance of life-situations or a surrender to a higher purpose, our ability to deal with some problems in everyone's life that cannot be easily solved is enhanced. Anger thus melts away.

Through the simple adjustments of diet recommended in this book (small meals and respect for good food combinations) that anyone can follow anytime, through the spine and breathing exercises and through overcoming fear and hurry for gain, acid reflux can effortlessly be banished once for all. Without any side effects. But there will be collateral benefits. Since all the various systems of the body are interconnected through the autonomic nervous system, improved health of the autonomic nervous system leads to improvements in blood glucose control, blood pressure, cholesterol and triglyceride levels, lower back pain, rheumatoid arthritis, asthma, eczema, allergies, skin tone and cardiovascular health.

(For more information on emotions and how they can be managed well, please refer to my book *5 Sheaths and One Self*.)

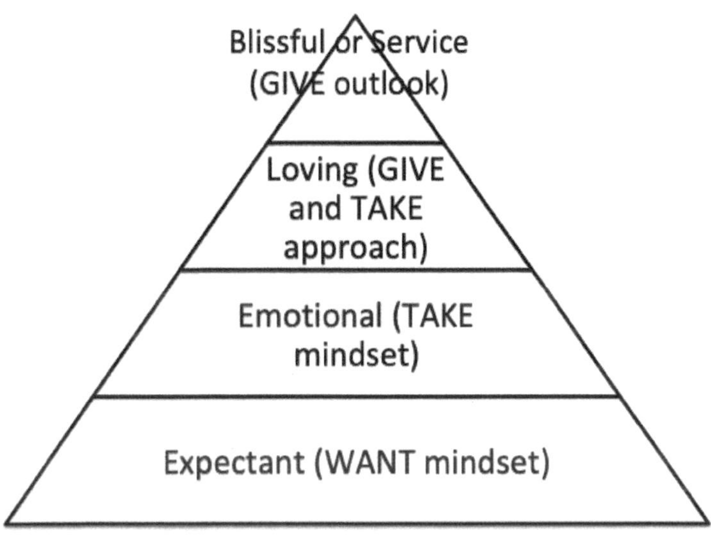



**The LOVE pyramid**

# 6 SOME THINGS TO REMEMBER

Here are some general tips for that would be helpful against acid reflux:

1.  Avoid tight-fitting clothes around the waist. The pressure on the stomach worsens reflux.
2.  Have small meals. After a meal, avoid bending forward while doing work or chores. Instead go down and up on your knees and sit on your haunches. This will not only avoid reflux but also back pain.
3.  If you are overweight, work on weight-reduction. In particular, extra weight around the waist exerts pressure on the stomach contents, worsening the heartburn.
4.  Do not take a shower immediately after a meal. This disturbs digestion.
5.  Avoid work that churns your stomach soon after a meal, again for the same reason. So, no vigorous exercise or brisk walking soon after a meal. A stroll after supper is recommended though for a good night's rest.
6.  Take a 15-minute break after lunch before resuming work. This keeps the stomach calm and retains energy levels.
7.  Avoid work after supper and restrict use of electronic gadgets. They affect the quality of sleep. Sound sleep is essential to keep reflux at bay.
8.  Avoid drinking water thirty minutes before a meal and two hours after it, and drink plenty at other times. This works

especially well if you have a leaky gut and tend to bloat after a meal.

9. Exercise should be done on an empty stomach or only at least 3-4 hours after a meal.
10. Eat only when hungry. Snacking in between meals or before a pervious meal is digested can damage health in the long run.
11. Drink milk and eat dairy products in moderation. Keep sugar consumption as low as possible.
12. Drink everyday your own homemade probiotic buttermilk (diluted yoghurt drink) with cooling spices like turmeric and cumin powder. For DIY yoghurt, add a spoon of yoghurt (with active bacterial culture) to a bowl of warm milk and leave it overnight. Your homemade yoghurt with a live culture will be ready in the morning.
13. Practise the exercise for emotional mastery in Chapter 4 regularly.
14. Eating habits should be regular. Regular routines and habits help in maintaining discipline and add to mental harmony. Irregular habits can lead to going off-limits and, as a consequence, can cause guilt.
15. Finally, don't worry and be happy. Everything will eventually work out. A study of the lives of most successful people will reveal how the odds were stacked against them at some point in their lives before things turned around.

# 7 EPILOGUE

Many of the ideas and concepts of this book have been drawn from traditional knowledge passed down through centuries in the form of Yoga and Ayurveda. That knowledge evolved and was developed when the concept of validation through randomized clinical trials did not exist. Nor was it formulated in the crucible of science and experimentation as we know it today. Yet, it stood the test of time and survived over centuries. And for a valid reason: simply because it worked.

I would call such traditional knowledge as an intuitive science because even though it seemingly did not evolve from an evidence-based approach, it still seems to work. How the ancient people discovered such sciences (and there are many such sciences) without the development of modern-day tools, methods and knowledge remains a mystery. In all likelihood, it must been revealed intuitively and perfected with practice. And the fact that a lot of it is increasingly passing the test of modern science (and, needless to add, individual experience) is reason enough to give it a try when everything else that we know of does not help.

# ABOUT THE AUTHOR

Bala Mookoni is a Life and Executive Coach. In Life Coaching, Mookoni covers Wellness, Weight Control, Emotional Competence, Relationships and Personal Goals. In Executive Coaching, he supports organizations in achieving Objectives, Performance and Productivity.

As every situation is unique, if the advice in this book has not worked for you, feel free to contact Mookoni at bala.mookoni@hilllakes.com or at +91 9904304232 to jointly work out other lifestyle adjustments that could help with your specific situation.